Gym Diary

Workout Log Book
With Food Planner / Diary

This Gym Diary Belongs To

_____

How To Use This Gym Diary

The diary is divided into two parts. On the right page, simply write the week beginning date at the top of the page and write everything down that you eat and drink on each day in that week. If you are counting your calories, you can write how many calories you consume each day too.

Summarize your week at the bottom of the page by writing about how you did overall. Anything that you want to write about your eating pattern, you put it in there.

The left page is for you to record your gym activity. Tracking your gym activity in this way is crucial as you will be able to see what you are doing and how this contributes to your overall fitness and health. It will become obvious what you need to do more of and also what is working well for you.

Write down the types of gym exercises and workouts that you do including the amount of sets and repetitions as you complete each one. In the notes section you can write a little bit about the impact of the individual exercises, your mood, your recovery after exercise, your water consumption, anything that you want to track.

Do not worry if you don't exercise every day, just fill this section out when you do with the date that you did the workout. (I bet you will not like to see this section blank and will exercise more just so you can fill it in). Summarize your week at the bottom of the page and track your fitness on a week by week basis.

This is your personal gym diary; it is a simple little diary for tracking a whole year's worth of workouts. By tracking your habits with this much detail you will become acutely aware of what you are eating and how serious you are taking your fitness goals.

This diary really gets under your skin and forces you to analyze yourself and make some positive changes in your life. So what are you waiting for? Get started today!

WEEKLY WORKOUT / FITNESS JOURNAL

Date	Exercise / Activity	Sets	Reps	Notes / Summary

Summary of my week

Weight

Food Journal

DATE	Breakfast	Lunch	Dinner	Snacks	Total
Mon					
Calories					
Tue					
Calories					
Wed					
Calories					
Thu					
Calories					
Fri					
Calories					
Sat					
Calories					
Sun					
Calories					

Summary of my week

WEEKLY WORKOUT / FITNESS JOURNAL

Date	Exercise / Activity	Sets	Reps	Notes / Summary

Summary of my week

Weight

Food Journal

DATE	Breakfast	Lunch	Dinner	Snacks	Total
Mon					
Calories					
Tue					
Calories					
Wed					
Calories					
Thu					
Calories					
Fri					
Calories					
Sat					
Calories					
Sun					
Calories					

Summary of my week

WEEKLY WORKOUT / FITNESS JOURNAL

Date	Exercise / Activity	Sets	Reps	Notes / Summary

Summary of my week

Weight

Food Journal

DATE	Breakfast	Lunch	Dinner	Snacks	Total
Mon					
Calories					
Tue					
Calories					
Wed					
Calories					
Thu					
Calories					
Fri					
Calories					
Sat					
Calories					
Sun					
Calories					

Summary of my week

WEEKLY WORKOUT / FITNESS JOURNAL

Date	Exercise / Activity	Sets	Reps	Notes / Summary

Summary of my week

Weight

Food Journal

DATE	Breakfast	Lunch	Dinner	Snacks	Total
Mon					
Calories					
Tue					
Calories					
Wed					
Calories					
Thu					
Calories					
Fri					
Calories					
Sat					
Calories					
Sun					
Calories					

Summary of my week

WEEKLY WORKOUT / FITNESS JOURNAL

Date	Exercise / Activity	Sets	Reps	Notes / Summary

Summary of my week

Weight

Food Journal

DATE	Breakfast	Lunch	Dinner	Snacks	Total
Mon					
Calories					
Tue					
Calories					
Wed					
Calories					
Thu					
Calories					
Fri					
Calories					
Sat					
Calories					
Sun					
Calories					

Summary of my week

WEEKLY WORKOUT / FITNESS JOURNAL

Date	Exercise / Activity	Sets	Reps	Notes / Summary

Summary of my week

Weight

Food Journal

DATE	Breakfast	Lunch	Dinner	Snacks	Total
Mon					
Calories					
Tue					
Calories					
Wed					
Calories					
Thu					
Calories					
Fri					
Calories					
Sat					
Calories					
Sun					
Calories					

Summary of my week

WEEKLY WORKOUT / FITNESS JOURNAL

Date	Exercise / Activity	Sets	Reps	Notes / Summary

Summary of my week

Weight

Food Journal

DATE	Breakfast	Lunch	Dinner	Snacks	Total
Mon					
Calories					
Tue					
Calories					
Wed					
Calories					
Thu					
Calories					
Fri					
Calories					
Sat					
Calories					
Sun					
Calories					

Summary of my week

WEEKLY WORKOUT / FITNESS JOURNAL

Date	Exercise / Activity	Sets	Reps	Notes / Summary

Summary of my week

Weight

Food Journal

DATE	Breakfast	Lunch	Dinner	Snacks	Total
Mon					
Calories					
Tue					
Calories					
Wed					
Calories					
Thu					
Calories					
Fri					
Calories					
Sat					
Calories					
Sun					
Calories					

Summary of my week

WEEKLY WORKOUT / FITNESS JOURNAL

Date	Exercise / Activity	Sets	Reps	Notes / Summary

Summary of my week

Weight

Food Journal

DATE	Breakfast	Lunch	Dinner	Snacks	Total
Mon					
Calories					
Tue					
Calories					
Wed					
Calories					
Thu					
Calories					
Fri					
Calories					
Sat					
Calories					
Sun					
Calories					

Summary of my week

WEEKLY WORKOUT / FITNESS JOURNAL

Date	Exercise / Activity	Sets	Reps	Notes / Summary

Summary of my week

Weight

Food Journal

DATE	Breakfast	Lunch	Dinner	Snacks	Total
Mon					
Calories					
Tue					
Calories					
Wed					
Calories					
Thu					
Calories					
Fri					
Calories					
Sat					
Calories					
Sun					
Calories					

Summary of my week

WEEKLY WORKOUT / FITNESS JOURNAL

Date	Exercise / Activity	Sets	Reps	Notes / Summary

Summary of my week

Weight

Food Journal

DATE	Breakfast	Lunch	Dinner	Snacks	Total
Mon					
Calories					
Tue					
Calories					
Wed					
Calories					
Thu					
Calories					
Fri					
Calories					
Sat					
Calories					
Sun					
Calories					

Summary of my week

WEEKLY WORKOUT / FITNESS JOURNAL

Date	Exercise / Activity	Sets	Reps	Notes / Summary

Summary of my week

Weight

Food Journal

DATE	Breakfast	Lunch	Dinner	Snacks	Total
Mon					
Calories					
Tue					
Calories					
Wed					
Calories					
Thu					
Calories					
Fri					
Calories					
Sat					
Calories					
Sun					
Calories					

Summary of my week

WEEKLY WORKOUT / FITNESS JOURNAL

Date	Exercise / Activity	Sets	Reps	Notes / Summary

Summary of my week

Weight

Food Journal

DATE	Breakfast	Lunch	Dinner	Snacks	Total
Mon					
Calories					
Tue					
Calories					
Wed					
Calories					
Thu					
Calories					
Fri					
Calories					
Sat					
Calories					
Sun					
Calories					

Summary of my week

WEEKLY WORKOUT / FITNESS JOURNAL

Date	Exercise / Activity	Sets	Reps	Notes / Summary

Summary of my week

Weight

Food Journal

DATE	Breakfast	Lunch	Dinner	Snacks	Total
Mon					
Calories					
Tue					
Calories					
Wed					
Calories					
Thu					
Calories					
Fri					
Calories					
Sat					
Calories					
Sun					
Calories					

Summary of my week

WEEKLY WORKOUT / FITNESS JOURNAL

Date	Exercise / Activity	Sets	Reps	Notes / Summary

Summary of my week

Weight

Food Journal

DATE	Breakfast	Lunch	Dinner	Snacks	Total
Mon					
Calories					
Tue					
Calories					
Wed					
Calories					
Thu					
Calories					
Fri					
Calories					
Sat					
Calories					
Sun					
Calories					

Summary of my week

WEEKLY WORKOUT / FITNESS JOURNAL

Date	Exercise / Activity	Sets	Reps	Notes / Summary

Summary of my week

Weight

Food Journal

DATE	Breakfast	Lunch	Dinner	Snacks	Total
Mon					
Calories					
Tue					
Calories					
Wed					
Calories					
Thu					
Calories					
Fri					
Calories					
Sat					
Calories					
Sun					
Calories					

Summary of my week

WEEKLY WORKOUT / FITNESS JOURNAL

Date	Exercise / Activity	Sets	Reps	Notes / Summary

Summary of my week

Weight

Food Journal

DATE	Breakfast	Lunch	Dinner	Snacks	Total
Mon					
Calories					
Tue					
Calories					
Wed					
Calories					
Thu					
Calories					
Fri					
Calories					
Sat					
Calories					
Sun					
Calories					

Summary of my week

WEEKLY WORKOUT / FITNESS JOURNAL

Date	Exercise / Activity	Sets	Reps	Notes / Summary

Summary of my week

Weight

Food Journal

DATE	Breakfast	Lunch	Dinner	Snacks	Total
Mon					
Calories					
Tue					
Calories					
Wed					
Calories					
Thu					
Calories					
Fri					
Calories					
Sat					
Calories					
Sun					
Calories					

Summary of my week

WEEKLY WORKOUT / FITNESS JOURNAL

Date	Exercise / Activity	Sets	Reps	Notes / Summary

Summary of my week

Weight

Food Journal

DATE	Breakfast	Lunch	Dinner	Snacks	Total
Mon					
Calories					
Tue					
Calories					
Wed					
Calories					
Thu					
Calories					
Fri					
Calories					
Sat					
Calories					
Sun					
Calories					

Summary of my week

WEEKLY WORKOUT / FITNESS JOURNAL

Date	Exercise / Activity	Sets	Reps	Notes / Summary

Summary of my week

Weight

Food Journal

DATE	Breakfast	Lunch	Dinner	Snacks	Total
Mon					
Calories					
Tue					
Calories					
Wed					
Calories					
Thu					
Calories					
Fri					
Calories					
Sat					
Calories					
Sun					
Calories					

Summary of my week

WEEKLY WORKOUT / FITNESS JOURNAL

Date	Exercise / Activity	Sets	Reps	Notes / Summary

Summary of my week

Weight

Food Journal

DATE	Breakfast	Lunch	Dinner	Snacks	Total
Mon					
Calories					
Tue					
Calories					
Wed					
Calories					
Thu					
Calories					
Fri					
Calories					
Sat					
Calories					
Sun					
Calories					

Summary of my week

WEEKLY WORKOUT / FITNESS JOURNAL

Date	Exercise / Activity	Sets	Reps	Notes / Summary

Summary of my week

Weight

Food Journal

DATE	Breakfast	Lunch	Dinner	Snacks	Total
Mon					
Calories					
Tue					
Calories					
Wed					
Calories					
Thu					
Calories					
Fri					
Calories					
Sat					
Calories					
Sun					
Calories					

Summary of my week

WEEKLY WORKOUT / FITNESS JOURNAL

Date	Exercise / Activity	Sets	Reps	Notes / Summary

Summary of my week

Weight

Food Journal

DATE	Breakfast	Lunch	Dinner	Snacks	Total
Mon					
Calories					
Tue					
Calories					
Wed					
Calories					
Thu					
Calories					
Fri					
Calories					
Sat					
Calories					
Sun					
Calories					

Summary of my week

WEEKLY WORKOUT / FITNESS JOURNAL

Date	Exercise / Activity	Sets	Reps	Notes / Summary

Summary of my week

Weight

Food Journal

DATE	Breakfast	Lunch	Dinner	Snacks	Total
Mon					
Calories					
Tue					
Calories					
Wed					
Calories					
Thu					
Calories					
Fri					
Calories					
Sat					
Calories					
Sun					
Calories					

Summary of my week

WEEKLY WORKOUT / FITNESS JOURNAL

Date	Exercise / Activity	Sets	Reps	Notes / Summary

Summary of my week

Weight

Food Journal

DATE	Breakfast	Lunch	Dinner	Snacks	Total
Mon					
Calories					
Tue					
Calories					
Wed					
Calories					
Thu					
Calories					
Fri					
Calories					
Sat					
Calories					
Sun					
Calories					

Summary of my week

WEEKLY WORKOUT / FITNESS JOURNAL

Date	Exercise / Activity	Sets	Reps	Notes / Summary

Summary of my week

Weight

Food Journal

DATE	Breakfast	Lunch	Dinner	Snacks	Total
Mon					
Calories					
Tue					
Calories					
Wed					
Calories					
Thu					
Calories					
Fri					
Calories					
Sat					
Calories					
Sun					
Calories					

Summary of my week

WEEKLY WORKOUT / FITNESS JOURNAL

Date	Exercise / Activity	Sets	Reps	Notes / Summary

Summary of my week

Weight

Food Journal

DATE	Breakfast	Lunch	Dinner	Snacks	Total
Mon					
Calories					
Tue					
Calories					
Wed					
Calories					
Thu					
Calories					
Fri					
Calories					
Sat					
Calories					
Sun					
Calories					

Summary of my week

WEEKLY WORKOUT / FITNESS JOURNAL

Date	Exercise / Activity	Sets	Reps	Notes / Summary

Summary of my week

Weight

Food Journal

DATE	Breakfast	Lunch	Dinner	Snacks	Total
Mon					
Calories					
Tue					
Calories					
Wed					
Calories					
Thu					
Calories					
Fri					
Calories					
Sat					
Calories					
Sun					
Calories					

Summary of my week

WEEKLY WORKOUT / FITNESS JOURNAL

Date	Exercise / Activity	Sets	Reps	Notes / Summary

Summary of my week

Weight

Food Journal

DATE	Breakfast	Lunch	Dinner	Snacks	Total
Mon					
Calories					
Tue					
Calories					
Wed					
Calories					
Thu					
Calories					
Fri					
Calories					
Sat					
Calories					
Sun					
Calories					

Summary of my week

WEEKLY WORKOUT / FITNESS JOURNAL

Date	Exercise / Activity	Sets	Reps	Notes / Summary

Summary of my week

Weight

Food Journal

DATE	Breakfast	Lunch	Dinner	Snacks	Total
Mon					
Calories					
Tue					
Calories					
Wed					
Calories					
Thu					
Calories					
Fri					
Calories					
Sat					
Calories					
Sun					
Calories					

Summary of my week

WEEKLY WORKOUT / FITNESS JOURNAL

Date	Exercise / Activity	Sets	Reps	Notes / Summary

Summary of my week

Weight

Food Journal

DATE	Breakfast	Lunch	Dinner	Snacks	Total
Mon					
Calories					
Tue					
Calories					
Wed					
Calories					
Thu					
Calories					
Fri					
Calories					
Sat					
Calories					
Sun					
Calories					

Summary of my week

WEEKLY WORKOUT / FITNESS JOURNAL

Date	Exercise / Activity	Sets	Reps	Notes / Summary

Summary of my week

Weight

Food Journal

DATE	Breakfast	Lunch	Dinner	Snacks	Total
Mon					
Calories					
Tue					
Calories					
Wed					
Calories					
Thu					
Calories					
Fri					
Calories					
Sat					
Calories					
Sun					
Calories					

Summary of my week

WEEKLY WORKOUT / FITNESS JOURNAL

Date	Exercise / Activity	Sets	Reps	Notes / Summary

Summary of my week

Weight

Food Journal

DATE	Breakfast	Lunch	Dinner	Snacks	Total
Mon					
Calories					
Tue					
Calories					
Wed					
Calories					
Thu					
Calories					
Fri					
Calories					
Sat					
Calories					
Sun					
Calories					

Summary of my week

WEEKLY WORKOUT / FITNESS JOURNAL

Date	Exercise / Activity	Sets	Reps	Notes / Summary

Summary of my week

Weight

Food Journal

DATE	Breakfast	Lunch	Dinner	Snacks	Total
Mon					
Calories					
Tue					
Calories					
Wed					
Calories					
Thu					
Calories					
Fri					
Calories					
Sat					
Calories					
Sun					
Calories					

Summary of my week

WEEKLY WORKOUT / FITNESS JOURNAL

Date	Exercise / Activity	Sets	Reps	Notes / Summary

Summary of my week

Weight

Food Journal

DATE	Breakfast	Lunch	Dinner	Snacks	Total
Mon					
Calories					
Tue					
Calories					
Wed					
Calories					
Thu					
Calories					
Fri					
Calories					
Sat					
Calories					
Sun					
Calories					

Summary of my week

WEEKLY WORKOUT / FITNESS JOURNAL

Date	Exercise / Activity	Sets	Reps	Notes / Summary

Summary of my week

Weight

Food Journal

DATE	Breakfast	Lunch	Dinner	Snacks	Total
Mon					
Calories					
Tue					
Calories					
Wed					
Calories					
Thu					
Calories					
Fri					
Calories					
Sat					
Calories					
Sun					
Calories					

Summary of my week

WEEKLY WORKOUT / FITNESS JOURNAL

Date	Exercise / Activity	Sets	Reps	Notes / Summary

Summary of my week

Weight

Food Journal

DATE	Breakfast	Lunch	Dinner	Snacks	Total
Mon					
Calories					
Tue					
Calories					
Wed					
Calories					
Thu					
Calories					
Fri					
Calories					
Sat					
Calories					
Sun					
Calories					

Summary of my week

WEEKLY WORKOUT / FITNESS JOURNAL

Date	Exercise / Activity	Sets	Reps	Notes / Summary

Summary of my week

Weight

Food Journal

DATE	Breakfast	Lunch	Dinner	Snacks	Total
Mon					
Calories					
Tue					
Calories					
Wed					
Calories					
Thu					
Calories					
Fri					
Calories					
Sat					
Calories					
Sun					
Calories					

Summary of my week

WEEKLY WORKOUT / FITNESS JOURNAL

Date	Exercise / Activity	Sets	Reps	Notes / Summary

Summary of my week

Weight

Food Journal

DATE	Breakfast	Lunch	Dinner	Snacks	Total
Mon					
Calories					
Tue					
Calories					
Wed					
Calories					
Thu					
Calories					
Fri					
Calories					
Sat					
Calories					
Sun					
Calories					

Summary of my week

WEEKLY WORKOUT / FITNESS JOURNAL

Date	Exercise / Activity	Sets	Reps	Notes / Summary

Summary of my week

Weight

Food Journal

DATE	Breakfast	Lunch	Dinner	Snacks	Total
Mon					
Calories					
Tue					
Calories					
Wed					
Calories					
Thu					
Calories					
Fri					
Calories					
Sat					
Calories					
Sun					
Calories					

Summary of my week

WEEKLY WORKOUT / FITNESS JOURNAL

Date	Exercise / Activity	Sets	Reps	Notes / Summary

Summary of my week

Weight

Food Journal

DATE	Breakfast	Lunch	Dinner	Snacks	Total
Mon					
Calories					
Tue					
Calories					
Wed					
Calories					
Thu					
Calories					
Fri					
Calories					
Sat					
Calories					
Sun					
Calories					

Summary of my week

WEEKLY WORKOUT / FITNESS JOURNAL

Date	Exercise / Activity	Sets	Reps	Notes / Summary

Summary of my week

Weight

Food Journal

DATE	Breakfast	Lunch	Dinner	Snacks	Total
Mon					
Calories					
Tue					
Calories					
Wed					
Calories					
Thu					
Calories					
Fri					
Calories					
Sat					
Calories					
Sun					
Calories					

Summary of my week

WEEKLY WORKOUT / FITNESS JOURNAL

Date	Exercise / Activity	Sets	Reps	Notes / Summary

Summary of my week

Weight

Food Journal

DATE	Breakfast	Lunch	Dinner	Snacks	Total
Mon					
Calories					
Tue					
Calories					
Wed					
Calories					
Thu					
Calories					
Fri					
Calories					
Sat					
Calories					
Sun					
Calories					

Summary of my week

WEEKLY WORKOUT / FITNESS JOURNAL

Date	Exercise / Activity	Sets	Reps	Notes / Summary

Summary of my week

Weight

Food Journal

DATE	Breakfast	Lunch	Dinner	Snacks	Total
Mon					
Calories					
Tue					
Calories					
Wed					
Calories					
Thu					
Calories					
Fri					
Calories					
Sat					
Calories					
Sun					
Calories					

Summary of my week

WEEKLY WORKOUT / FITNESS JOURNAL

Date	Exercise / Activity	Sets	Reps	Notes / Summary

Summary of my week

Weight

Food Journal

DATE	Breakfast	Lunch	Dinner	Snacks	Total
Mon					
Calories					
Tue					
Calories					
Wed					
Calories					
Thu					
Calories					
Fri					
Calories					
Sat					
Calories					
Sun					
Calories					

Summary of my week

WEEKLY WORKOUT / FITNESS JOURNAL

Date	Exercise / Activity	Sets	Reps	Notes / Summary

Summary of my week

Weight

Food Journal

DATE	Breakfast	Lunch	Dinner	Snacks	Total
Mon					
Calories					
Tue					
Calories					
Wed					
Calories					
Thu					
Calories					
Fri					
Calories					
Sat					
Calories					
Sun					
Calories					

Summary of my week

WEEKLY WORKOUT / FITNESS JOURNAL

Date	Exercise / Activity	Sets	Reps	Notes / Summary

Summary of my week

Weight

Food Journal

DATE	Breakfast	Lunch	Dinner	Snacks	Total
Mon					
Calories					
Tue					
Calories					
Wed					
Calories					
Thu					
Calories					
Fri					
Calories					
Sat					
Calories					
Sun					
Calories					

Summary of my week

WEEKLY WORKOUT / FITNESS JOURNAL

Date	Exercise / Activity	Sets	Reps	Notes / Summary

Summary of my week

Weight

Food Journal

DATE	Breakfast	Lunch	Dinner	Snacks	Total
Mon					
Calories					
Tue					
Calories					
Wed					
Calories					
Thu					
Calories					
Fri					
Calories					
Sat					
Calories					
Sun					
Calories					

Summary of my week

WEEKLY WORKOUT / FITNESS JOURNAL

Date	Exercise / Activity	Sets	Reps	Notes / Summary

Summary of my week

Weight

Food Journal

DATE	Breakfast	Lunch	Dinner	Snacks	Total
Mon					
Calories					
Tue					
Calories					
Wed					
Calories					
Thu					
Calories					
Fri					
Calories					
Sat					
Calories					
Sun					
Calories					

Summary of my week

WEEKLY WORKOUT / FITNESS JOURNAL

Date	Exercise / Activity	Sets	Reps	Notes / Summary

Summary of my week

Weight

Food Journal

DATE	Breakfast	Lunch	Dinner	Snacks	Total
Mon					
Calories					
Tue					
Calories					
Wed					
Calories					
Thu					
Calories					
Fri					
Calories					
Sat					
Calories					
Sun					
Calories					

Summary of my week

WEEKLY WORKOUT / FITNESS JOURNAL

Date	Exercise / Activity	Sets	Reps	Notes / Summary

Summary of my week

Weight

Food Journal

DATE	Breakfast	Lunch	Dinner	Snacks	Total
Mon					
Calories					
Tue					
Calories					
Wed					
Calories					
Thu					
Calories					
Fri					
Calories					
Sat					
Calories					
Sun					
Calories					

Summary of my week

WEEKLY WORKOUT / FITNESS JOURNAL

Date	Exercise / Activity	Sets	Reps	Notes / Summary

Summary of my week

Weight

Food Journal

DATE	Breakfast	Lunch	Dinner	Snacks	Total
Mon					
Calories					
Tue					
Calories					
Wed					
Calories					
Thu					
Calories					
Fri					
Calories					
Sat					
Calories					
Sun					
Calories					

Summary of my week

Need another gym diary?
Visit www.blankboksnjournals.com

14362351R00060

Printed in Great Britain
by Amazon